STEP WORKBOOK FOR

ADOLESCENT CHEMICAL DEPENDENCY RECOVERY

A GUIDE TO THE FIRST FIVE STEPS

AF713871

BY STEVEN L. JAFFE, M.D.

AMERICAN ACADEMY OF CHILD & ADOLESCENT PSYCHIATRY
AACAP
1953

NAME ______________________________

STEP WORKBOOK FOR

ADOLESCENT CHEMICAL DEPENDENCY RECOVERY

A GUIDE TO THE FIRST FIVE STEPS

BY STEVEN L. JAFFE, M.D.

NAME ______________________________

Books published by the American Academy of Child & Adolescent Psychiatry represent the views and opinions of the individual authors and do not necessarily represent the policies and opinions of the Academy.

Copyright © 1990 American Academy of Child and Adolescent Psychiatry

ALL RIGHTS RESERVED

Manufactured in the United States of America

06 05 04 03 02   14 13 12 11 10

ISBN 1-882103-00-9

Distributed by the American Psychiatric Press, Inc.
1400 K Street, N.W., Washington, DC 20005

Library of Congress Cataloging-in-Publication Data

Jaffe, Steven L., 1940-
The step workbook for adolescent chemical dependency recovery : a guide to the first five steps / Steven L. Jaffe.
p. cm.
Summary: A guide for teenagers to work the first five steps of a twelve step program as part of a chemical dependency treatment program.
ISBN 1-882103-00-9
1. Alcoholics Anonymous—Juvenile literature. 2. Alcoholism—Treatment—Juvenile literature. 3. Alcoholics—Rehabiltation—Juvenile literature. 4. Teenagers—Alcohol use—Juvenile literature. [1. Drug abuse—Treatment. 2. Alcoholism—Treatment. 3. Substance abuse—Treatment.] I. American Academy of Child and Adolescent Psychiatry. II. Title.
HV5066.J34 1990
362.29'286'0835—dc20

Contents

About the Author

Steven L. Jaffe, M.D. received his psychiatry training at Harvard University and the Massachusetts Mental Health Center, and his child psychiatry training at Emory University. He has been Editor of the Newsletter of the American Academy of Child and Adolescent Psychiatry and President of the Georgia Council for Child and Adolescent Psychiatry. Dr. Jaffe is currently the Director of Adolescent Programs, Psychiatric and Chemical Dependency, at CPC-Parkwood Hospital and Associate Professor of Child and Adolescent Psychiatry at Emory University in Atlanta, Georgia.

Acknowledgments

I am grateful to the following individuals for their help in preparing this workbook:

LeNora M. Ashley, M.D.
Susan Tucker, M.S.
Roanne Jaffe, M.Ed.
Randy Johnson
G. Ashley Kilpatrick

Introduction

[T]o sustain a single human soul is equivalent to sustaining an entire world.

—Talmud

This workbook has been developed to aid and correctly structure a teenager's working the first five steps of Alcoholics Anonymous and Narcotics Anonymous. This workbook has been developed as part of a multimodality treatment program of which the Twelve Steps of AA/NA are a fundamental part. Because chemically dependent teenagers frequently have school and learning problems, these exercises have been written at an easier reading and understanding level.

How to Use *The Step Workbook*

This copy of *The Step Workbook for Adolescent Chemical Dependency Recovery* belongs to *you*. This is your special place to write down your thoughts, your feelings, and your secrets. No one else will read what you have written until you show this workbook to them. For this workbook to be helpful, remember the following advice:

- *Go ahead and write on the pages.* This is your personal copy of the workbook. It doesn't matter whether you use pencil, pen, or marker. No one will "grade" your answers. Spelling doesn't count. This workbook is a place for you to organize your thoughts and feelings and to express them clearly on paper.
- *Use extra paper if you need to.* For many of the questions, we have provided some space for you to write directly in the book. But you might want to write more than will fit in the available space. Keep some extra paper handy to use when you want to write more. If you copy the workbook page number and question number on any extra sheets you use, you will be able to keep track of your answers when you want to go back and read them.
- *Interact with others.* Step 1 and your life history will be presented and discussed at specific groups. Steps 2 and 3 will be discussed individually with staff and may be discussed at groups.
- *Step 4 is special.* In Step 4 you will be writing down the most personal secrets from your life. Write down the answers on separate paper, using as much space as you need. In Step 5, you will be telling these answers to someone you trust to keep your secrets. If you like, after you have completed Step 5, you can tear up your answers to the questions from Step 4 and throw them away. You might want to keep the rest of the workbook to read as you rework these steps in the future.
- *Don't rush.* There is no hurry to complete this workbook. Complete one section at a time.
- *Ask questions.* If you don't understand a question in the workbook, skip that question and go back to it later. Don't be afraid to ask for help in reading and understanding the questions. No one should give you help in writing the answers, though, since it's important that the answers be yours alone.
- *Be honest with yourself.* The most important part of this workbook is facing your problems honestly. When you answer the workbook questions, writing lies and denying the truth will simply delay your recovery. This is a very special opportunity for you to make an important change in your life. You owe it to yourself to stop the lies and find the truth.
- *Don't be afraid of your emotions.* Many of the issues brought up in the workbook will cause you to feel some very strong emotions: sadness, panic, anxiety, shame, or rage. Don't try to avoid these reactions. They are a normal part of facing these issues and being honest with yourself. If the emotions are strong,

talk to staff about the memories and feelings. And, as you continue to write in the workbook, you will probably experience some new emotions growing: relief and better feelings about yourself.

- *Be willing to accept the help of others.* The staff members and the other teenagers in your group will discuss your answers to the questions in the workbook. They will keep these discussions confidential, and they will help you make the first five steps toward freedom from chemical dependency.

The Twelve Steps of Alcoholics Anonymous

The Twelve Steps to recovery are as follows:

1. We admitted we were powerless over alcohol—that our lives had become unmanageable.
2. Came to believe that a Power greater than ourselves could restore us to sanity.
3. Made a decision to turn our will and our lives over to the care of God as we understand Him.
4. Made a searching and fearless moral inventory of ourselves.
5. Admitted to God, to ourselves, and to another human being the exact nature of our wrongs.
6. Were entirely ready to have God remove all these defects of character.
7. Humbly asked Him to remove our shortcomings.
8. Made a list of all persons we had harmed, and became willing to make amends to them all.
9. Made direct amends to such people wherever possible, except when to do so would injure them or others.
10. Continued to take personal inventory and when we were wrong promptly admitted it.
11. Sought through prayer and meditation to improve our conscious contact with God as we understood Him, praying only for knowledge of His will for us and the power to carry that out.
12. Having had a spiritual awakening as the result of these steps, we tried to carry this message to alcoholics, and to practice these principles in all our affairs.

Author's note: This workbook is our interpretation of a guide for adolescents in hospital or residential recovery programs to work the first five Steps. The Steps are adapted with permission, and the opinions expressed are those of the authors. This workbook does not officially speak for any Twelve Step organization.

Source: The Twelve Steps are taken from Alcoholics Anonymous (Third Edition), published by A.A. World Services, Inc., New York, NY, pp. 59–60. Reprinted with permission.

Screening: Some Basics of Drug Use

	Check if you have done this	How often (every day, number of times per week)?	For how long?
Pot (Marijuana)	______	______	______
Acid (LSD)	______	______	______
Uppers (stimulants)	______	______	______
Downers (barbiturates, Quaaludes)	______	______	______
Coke (cocaine, crack, ice)	______	______	______
Alcohol	______	______	______
Glue, gasoline, Freon (inhalants/huffing)	______	______	______
My favorite drug is ______	______	______	______

Some key questions:

	Yes	No
1. Do you cut school and then drink or use drugs?	________	________
2. Have you ever stolen anything to support your drinking/using?	________	________
3. Have you ever sold drugs?	________	________
4. Do you drink until you are drunk?	________	________
5. Have you ever been in trouble with the police due to drinking or using?	________	________
6. Have you ever experienced a blackout? (A blackout is when you wake up from having passed out and you don't remember what others said you did.)	________	________
7. Is there alcoholism and/or drug abuse in any of your family members?	________	________
8. Have you ever sneaked out at night in order to get high?	________	________
9. Have you ever lied to your parents or other people about your drinking or drug use?	________	________
10. Have you missed school because of drinking or drugs?	________	________

Step 1

We admitted we were powerless over alcohol (or drugs)—that our lives had become unmanageable.

Let's see how much you've lost because of drugs or alcohol.

How? By completing the First Step and admitting the truth.

Fill in these pages. It's time to stop lying and to *get honest* with yourself.

Step 1: Inventory

You have been admitted to a treatment program for drug or alcohol problems, and you aren't sure whether you need to be here. You may admit that you use "a little." But you're not out of control. Well . . . let's see. The purpose of Step 1 is for you to write down your problem and face how serious it is.

Be honest!!

This is a special opportunity. It could mean life or death. Don't waste your time with lies. Write the truth and let's look at whether you have a problem.

Risk Taking

1. Write about the times drugs or alcohol have put your life in danger.

2. Did you risk the lives of others when you were using drugs or alcohol?

3. Have you ever thought about killing yourself? Explain.

Thinking Less of Yourself

1. What have you done sexually when you were high that you wished you had not done?

2. Write about the times when someone has hurt you physically or the times when you have hurt others (being beaten up, rape, gang fights, etc.).

3. What things have you done to get drugs or while on drugs that you told yourself you would *never* do?

Breaking the Law

1. Give examples of times you have broken the law while using drugs or while trying to get money to use (shoplifting, stealing money or cars, prostitution, etc.).

2. Tell about the times you were arrested, sent to jail or juvenile court, or just "picked up" by the police.

3. Did you deal drugs or alcohol? ______ Yes ______ No. Where and to what age groups?

4. Have you ever used a false ID to buy alcohol or asked an adult to buy it for you? ______ Yes ______ No.

5. How many times have you skipped school to use alcohol or drugs?
______ Once or twice ______ Many times.

6. How many times have you missed school because you were too sick from alcohol or drugs (hung over, hadn't been to bed yet, etc.)?
______ Once or twice ______ Many times.

7. Have you ever been suspended from school? ______ Yes ______ No. Why?

8. Did your grades or school participation go down because of drugs?
______ Yes ______ No. Describe what happened:

9. Did you ever drink or use drugs on school grounds? ______ Yes ______ No.

Losing the Trust of Your Family

1. What behaviors does your family complain about the most?

2. Did your family know about your drug or alcohol problem?
______ Yes ______ No ______ I'm not sure.

3. Have you ever done these things? *(Put a check next to the ones you've done.)*
______ a. Tried to sneak out at night to get high.
______ b. Used drugs or alcohol at home.
______ c. Stolen money from family to buy drugs or alcohol.
______ d. Used drugs and then lied to parents about it.

Issues with Friends

1. Before you began using or drinking, did you have "straight" friends?
______ Yes ______ No. What things did you do with them for fun?

2. Write about the friends you have now. Are they drug users, straight, etc.?

3. a. If you still have straight friends, do they know that you use?

   b. What do they say or think about your drug or alcohol use?

4. a. What things did you do for fun that you don't do anymore because of your drug or alcohol use?

   b. Why did you stop doing them (don't have time, too messed up to do it, drug friends don't think it's "cool," etc.)?

5. Do you think you are part of the drug culture or group? ______ Yes ______ No. Why or why not?

6. What did most people at your school (or neighborhood) think about you? (What was your "image"?)

Effect on Your Body and Brain

1. Put a check by the problems you have had because of drug or alcohol use. Describe when the problem began, how often it occurs, and how much it bothers you.

   _____ a. Trouble with memory (blackouts, can't remember things in school, can't pay attention, etc.).

   _____ b. Getting dizzy.

   _____ c. Having flashbacks or seeing trails.

   _____ d. Hands, feet, or legs getting numb.

   _____ e. Trouble sleeping.

   _____ f. Getting the shakes ("nerves") if you try to stay off drugs or alcohol.

______ g. Don't care about doing anything.

Running Away from Painful Feelings

Sometimes you may drink or get high to escape from painful feelings of sadness or anxiety. Write about these feelings and what caused them.

Effects on Your Mind

1. Write about the times you were thinking about drugs or alcohol (or how to get them) when you were supposed to be thinking about school, work, or people.

2. Give examples of things (like homework or chores) you forgot to do because you were high or drunk.

3. Have you ever tried to control how much you used drugs or alcohol ("I'll just smoke one joint," or "I'll just have one drink," or "I won't use anything tonight.")? ______ Yes ______ No.

4. Write about some of the times you ended up using or drinking too much anyway and couldn't stop.

Giving Up Plans for the Future

1. If you had not come into this program now, what would have happened to you?

2. Before you started using or drinking, what plans and goals did you have for your life?

3. How did your plans and goals change after you began using?

Summary

Addicts are people who, once they use a drug, have to keep using even though their life is a mess and getting worse. They no longer care about school, job, family, or friends. They will lie, cheat, and steal to get drugs. The First Step is for you to see whether you are an addict or if you are on the way to becoming an addict.

1. Do your answers to any of the questions help you see that your life is a mess because of drugs? ______ Yes ______ No, not really. Which questions?

2. Can you accept that you are an alcoholic or drug addict? ______ Yes ______ No ______ Not sure—maybe I'm on the way to becoming an addict.

3. Many confess that they have no control over their drug use, but they don't really believe it. What would it take to make you believe you are powerless over using alcohol or drugs?

4. What about your life is most like an addict's life?

5. Name things you could change (in a good way) about your life while in this program.

6. Filling out these First Step questions could be just a joke, unless you have been totally ________.

Now you will present your First Step inventory to a
First Step group so you can hear your own thoughts and get feedback.

Take the risk of being honest!

Your life depends on it!

Your Life History

Now you are about to write about your life. You need to make some sense of your life—to begin to put some of the pieces together so you can begin to feel whole.

This will help you to understand what you caused to happen and what was out of your control. Sometimes as a child you blame yourself for things you couldn't change.

"What's the best way to get this done?"

1. *Just start!!* Get in there and do it. Don't wait until you're "in the mood."

2. *Do one or two parts at a time.* If you try to do the whole life story all at once, you may feel overwhelmed.

3. *Write down the facts and the feelings.* We want to know how you felt about the things that happened to you.

Try not to worry about "how it sounds," what your peers will think, or whether anyone will still like you. You'll be scared to tell some of your secrets, but so is everyone.

You will probably find out that you are not very different from others in the program.

Everyone has done stupid
or cruel things in their life
and
everyone has had stupid
or cruel things done to them.

You are not alone and there is no reason to be embarrassed or afraid.

Be honest about your whole life, not just your alcohol and drug use. If you keep secrets inside, they make you sick.

Get them out and get free!

A. Childhood

1. When and where were you born?

2. What did people say you were like as a baby (easy, difficult, hyper or overly sensitive)?

3. Describe your strongest memories as a young child:

4. Describe your childhood friends:

5. Games you remember playing:

6. Describe happy times as a child:

7. Describe "horrible" scary times (such as physical or sexual abuse, accidents, hospitalizations, etc.):

8. Write about some sad experiences:

B. Family Relationships

1. Who is in your family and what is each person like?

2. How do you get along with each member of your family?

3. Write about what serious problems your family has had (death, suicide attempts, long hospital stays for physical or emotional problems, alcoholism or drug abuse):

4. Are your parents divorced? ______ Yes ______ No.
   If Yes, who do you live with?

   What is it like to have a stepparent?

   Do you get caught between your parents' anger at each other?

5. Is your family getting better or worse? Explain.

6. What does your family do for fun?

7. What did your parents do when you did something wrong (talk to you, hit you, beat you)?

8. How did your parents respond when you did something well?

9. Describe who was the "real boss" in your family—the person who made the decisions and directed the family?

C. School

1. Your grades in elementary school:

   middle school:

   high school:

2. Behavior (shy, class clown, arguments and fights) in elementary school:

   middle school:

   high school:

   Did your grades or behavior change after you began using alcohol or drugs? ______ Yes ______ No. If yes, describe what happened.

3. Do you have a reading or learning problem? ______ Yes ______ No. If yes, describe it:

4. Were you in special education classes? ______ Yes ______ No.
   If Yes, how did you feel about this?

5. Write about any special awards and accomplishments (honor roll, sports, etc.):

6. Were you ever suspended? ______ Yes ______ No. If yes, why?

   Were you ever sent to the principal or a counselor for discipline problems? ______ Yes ______ No. If yes, why?

7. What were your friends like in
   elementary school:

   middle school:

   high school:

D. Legal Problems

List what you did that was illegal even if you didn't get caught:

1.

2.

3.

4.

5.

6.

7.

8.

Circle the numbers of the things you did to get money for alcohol or drugs. Write an X next to the things you did before drugs.

E. Treatment

1. What did you do to be put in this program?

2. How do you feel about being here?

3. What are you learning?

F. Future

1. What about you still needs to be changed?

2. What's OK or good about you?

3. What are your plans for discharge and aftercare?

4. In one year, where do you hope to be and what will you be doing?

G. Summary

The First Step helps you to admit that you were powerless over drugs and alcohol. Now that you have looked back on your life, what other things have you been powerless over? Describe those things in your life you wished were different, but you couldn't change (having to move to a different city, parents getting a divorce, a parent using alcohol or drugs, someone dying, being abused, etc.).

Have you felt guilty that you should have changed these things?
______ Yes ______ No. How have you tried to change some of these things?

Do you think that when you're an adult, you'll have more control over things? Why or why not?

Now you will share your life story with the group.

Step 2

Came to believe that a Power greater than ourselves could restore us to sanity.

"I can't change by myself."

"I need some help!"

Step 2 involves first examining whether your addict behavior is irrational and self-destructive. If you keep doing something that makes you feel bad and risks your life, it's nonsense to keep doing it. The second part involves needing something positive and good beyond yourself.

Part 1: Senseless Behavior

1. Check the things that happened as a result of your drinking or drug-using behavior:

A	B
____ Got busted or arrested	____ Grades went up
____ Had an accident	____ Family acted nice to me
____ Got hassled by parents	____ Made straight friends
____ Was suspended from school	____ Saved money for a car, college, etc.
____ Physically hurt someone	____ Most people trusted me
____ Got pregnant or got someone pregnant	____ Did well in sports, band, clubs, etc.
____ Grades went down	____ Parents were proud of me—we got along well
____ Lost a friend	____ Was able to have a part-time job and still do well in school
____ Got parents upset	
____ Got others hooked on drugs or alcohol	
____ Got placed in a treatment program	
____ Was physically hurt (raped, beaten, etc.)	

How many "B" answers do you have? ______

How many "A" answers do you have? ______

So how was your life going? If you:

1) had more "B" answers, "Then, why are you here?"
2) had more "A" answers, ". . . and *you* said you drank or used for *fun*?"

2. Which of these things could have happened because of your behavior while using or drinking?:

____ a. I could have been killed or seriously injured in a car accident (or killed or injured others in the car).

____ b. I could have been put into juvenile detention or jail.

____ c. I could have "passed out"/"blacked out" in a dangerous place or time.

____ d. I could have been kicked out of the house by my parents.

____ e. I could have caused serious damage to my body (heart attack from cocaine, heart or liver disease from alcohol).

____ f. I could have been killed or seriously injured by someone in a fight.

____ g. I could have attempted suicide if I had gone on long enough.

Circle the letter(s) of the things above that *have already happened* to you.

Alcohol and drugs made you feel high and not care. As an addict, you couldn't moderate the use of alcohol or drugs, and irrational self-destructive behavior was repeated over and over. Your way hasn't worked.

Part 2: A Higher Power

Using a higher power involves believing and trusting in something positive beyond yourself.

As a young child, who were your higher powers (a parent, older brother or sister, aunt or uncle, etc.)?

Did your childhood higher powers ever hurt you or let you down?
____ Yes ____ No. If yes, describe what happened and describe how you felt?

When and how did you begin to mistrust the authority figures in your life?

When did you see these authority figures as "the enemy" and decide that "your way" was the only way?

When you were heavily using drugs or alcohol, you developed specific beliefs about yourself and the world. (Check which of the following you believed. You can mark more than one.)

____ a. It's OK to tell lies.

____ b. You can live without any pain or distress.

____ c. If it feels good, it is good.

____ d. Do whatever it takes to get what you want.

____ e. Authority figures (parents, teachers, police, clergy) are the enemy.

____ f. Your way is the only way.

____ g. Straight people don't really care and only want you to be miserable like them.

____ h. You can only trust "using" friends.

____ i. You can take what you want.

These beliefs made you feel strong and in control. The problem is these beliefs just are *not* true and *don't* work. Why is it so difficult to accept that these beliefs have not worked?

Your First Step and part 1 of Step 2 prove that these specific beliefs don't work. Now you need to find a belief system that is true and does work.

1. How do you feel about depending on (or believing in) a higher power? (You may mark more than one.)

____ a. Forget it! I didn't come here to become a religious freak.

____ b. I've already tried it, but it didn't work. God has never answered my prayers or helped me out of a hole before.

____ c. I believe in God.

____ d. I don't depend on anyone and no one tells me what to do.

____ e. I hope there's something that can help me straighten out my life.

____ f. I couldn't believe in a higher power—you can't prove that one exists.

____ g. I'm not sure—it's confusing.

____ h. Other. I feel ____

____

____

2. You can choose to think of a higher power in many different ways. Below are some of the higher powers that other people have used. Mark the one that you think might work for you. (You may mark more than one.)

____ a. God/Jesus/Buddha/Mohammed.

____ b. AA or NA.

____ c. "the group" you are in treatment with.

____ d. "the program."

____ e. a warm feeling you've had during good times in your life.

____ f. a sponsor (for awhile).

____ g. a "made up" or ideal parent.

____ h. the energy of the world (a positive supernatural force, a power source).

____ i. the Twelve Steps.

____ j. an invisible or "made up" friend—a "partner."

____ k. "something" you know is there but you can't describe.

____ l. other (explain) ____

____

____

Being restored to sanity implies being able to do what one *needs* to do and not what one *wants* to do. One needs to be sane and abstinent from alcohol and drugs. This requires becoming honest and caring about yourself and others. Beginning to believe that there is something positive beyond oneself to help in this process is what Step 2 involves.

At AA/NA meetings, you will see other addicts who have thought and acted the way you have. Seeing that they have found a positive higher power will help you believe that a life without alcohol and drugs is possible.

People that you meet who are in Twelve Step programs (staff, volunteers, members of AA/NA, contacts) have developed a new belief system with a positive higher power. Check which of the following beliefs you have noticed in these people:

____ a. Be honest to yourself and others.

____ b. Be responsible for what you do and don't do.

____ c. Pain and distress are a part of life.

____ d. Tolerate the sadness of losses and disappointments.

____ e. Authority figures care enough to say "no."

____ f. Respect and care about other people.

____ g. Recognize and tolerate your feelings.

____ h. Living *without* drugs or alcohol gives you the power to have a life and future.

Circle which of the above beliefs you might agree with. Which ones are the most important?

Can you begin to believe that there is something positive which will help you? ____ Yes ____ No ____ Not sure ____ Maybe.

Now you will discuss this step individually with a staff member.

Step 3

Made a decision to turn our will and our lives over to the care of God as we understand Him.

The Third Step involves the development of a decision to commit yourself to a positive spiritual higher power.

In this step, you learn to "turn over"—this means you place those uncontrollable parts of your life into the care of a higher power. This allows you to put your energies into what you can control (your behavior), and leaves other issues (what your fathers, mothers, and others do or don't do) up to a higher power.

In the First Step you faced that your uncontrollable alcohol or drug use became a self-destructive, meaningless way of life. The Second Step involved beginning to believe that something positive beyond yourself could move you to an honest life without alcohol or drugs. In the Third Step, you start that new way of thinking, feeling, and acting.

Accepting that you are an addict (chemically dependent) means that you accept that there are incidents and people in your life that you couldn't and can't control. Describe the most painful event in your life that you couldn't control (i.e., parents getting divorced, being rejected by someone you loved, being raped or abused).

You used alcohol or drugs to try to avoid the pain of events like this. Circle which feelings you tried to deny.

ANGER	FEAR	ANXIETY	INADEQUACY
SADNESS	LONELINESS	INFERIORITY	BOREDOM

Now, put a * in front of the feeling you have the most trouble tolerating.

Alcohol and drugs made you numb, and you could pretend you were cool and didn't care. You desperately tried to control your life. The reality of addiction eventually intervened. Now it's scary to admit that what you were so sure of, so dedicated to, didn't work. Check what you might be afraid of in giving up old ways. Describe your thoughts and feelings.

______ 1. Admitting you don't have the answers.

______ 2. Admitting you were really weak under your tough image.

______ 3. Admitting you are *not* unique and different from everyone else.

Now comes the challenge of trying a different way. Pretend you injured your ankle. It swelled and was quite painful. You put ice on it and elevated the leg, but the pain got worse. You pretended it didn't hurt much and tried to walk on it. This didn't work. The pain became intolerable and the ankle became so weak you couldn't even stand up. Finally, you feel desperate. You've done everything you can think of to control the pain and strengthen the ankle, but you can't manage it on your own. You go to a doctor to see if something can be done. The doctor recommends surgery because of damaged tendons. You now have a choice (check one):

______ 1. You can turn down the surgery and keep trying to do it on your own, or
______ 2. You can make a decision to have the treatment.

This is what Step 3 involves:
Agreeing to be treated.

The treatment will involve some discomfort and pain, and specific instructions of what you must do and not do to allow the ankle to recover. You don't automatically feel better when you agree to the treatment. You make the decision to follow the directions and guidance of a new way of thinking, feeling, and acting. Here you learn to "turn it over."

You previously "turned over" your life to alcohol or drugs. Describe what this was like for you:

Did you go to any length to get what you wanted?
______ Yes ______ Sometimes ______ Never.

Now you are going to commit to a positive way of life.

You are not going to trust everybody because you know there are people actively using alcohol or drugs who may hurt you. Here you are committing to a set of positive principles rather than your own will.

What are you afraid of in trying a new way (for example, fear of the unknown without your security blanket of drugs, feeling you won't be able to do it differently)? Describe your fears:

Making this decision doesn't mean you feel better, only that you will take a journey to be better.

As a child, did you believe in anything positive beyond yourself (a mother or father, relative, stuffed animal, church, nature, beautiful sunset, God)? Describe what you believed:

How did this belief make you feel?

Was there a point in your life when you stopped believing (when and why)?

Describe your idea of God:

Many teenagers feel that the God part is too much to believe in and use this as an excuse not to work the program. If this applies to you, try thinking of it as a "good orderly direction."

Giving up the alcohol or drug use which you were powerless to manage and committing yourself to a positive higher power will give you a new sense of peace and the power to live a good life.

Now you will discuss this step with staff.

Step 4

Made a searching and fearless moral inventory of ourselves.

Step 4: Inventory

You are now ready to look back at every part of your life to see what kind of person you have been and what has made you the way you are. You will be writing down all the things you have done or felt in your life.

Unless you get rid of your fears, guilt, and hates, they will stay with you and cause pain. Then you'll have to take a "pain reliever" (alcohol or drugs) again. You must let yourself remember in order to leave the pain behind.

Write down everything that has been painful or embarrassing or has filled you with anger or shame. Be as honest and complete as you can. Be sure to put down all the positive things that have happened to you and the good points about yourself.

Remember: You are as sick as your secrets.

In Step 4, you are going to write about every good and bad action, thought, and feeling you can remember. Frequently, remembering these issues causes anxieties, sadness, and rage to be reexperienced. Don't panic—this is a normal part of doing a Fourth Step. It means you are working hard, being honest, and remembering painful issues.

My Early Life and My Family Life

1. What were you told or know about your birth? Were you planned, were you wanted, or were you a surprise?
2. What do you know about your family's situation when you were an infant? Write about what number child you were, money problems, relatives living in the household, and any other difficulties in the family while you were an infant.
3. Who were you named after and what does that mean to you?
4. Were you an only child?
5. What do you know about whether your parents wanted you to be a boy or girl, and what did they communicate to you about this? Did they dress you or treat you as if you were the opposite sex?
6. Did you have brothers and sisters? How old were you when your younger siblings were born? What feelings and memories do you have about them when they were born and as you were growing up?
7. What were you told about yourself when you were a toddler (two years old)? Were you considered difficult, hyper, or prone to many temper tantrums?
8. When you were a child, was your mother or father sick and was either in the hospital?
9. What do you remember about whether the family was troubled or happy? Did you spend periods of time away from your family?
10. Were you moved around to different relatives or with a foster family?
11. Why do you think this occurred?
12. How were you punished? Were you spanked, whipped, sent to your room, or did you have things taken away?
13. How did you feel when you were punished (did you feel hatred; did you feel degraded)?
14. Did you have chores and jobs to do around the house? Did you do them?
15. Did you feel loved and wanted or did you feel rejected and abandoned as a young child?
16. In your family who was your mother's favorite child and who was your father's favorite child? How did this make you feel?
17. Did your family praise you and tell you that you were a good person?
18. How did your parents react when you felt lonely or sad?
19. What did you do to get your family's attention?
20. Were you babied and overprotected by your mother or father? How did they do this and how did you feel?
21. Were you spoiled? Did your parents shield you from the consequences of your behavior?
22. As a young child, do you remember hating your mother or father? Why do you think you felt this?

23. As a young child, what do you remember about how your mother and father treated each other? Were they affectionate, loving, caring, or neutral to each other, or did they argue and seem to hate each other?
24. When your parents argued or fought, how did this make you feel (scared, angry)?
25. Did you side with one parent against the other? Which parent? How did this make you feel?
26. Did you feel that you had a place in the family or did you feel left out?
27. What is your religion? How religious was your family? How was this taught to you and how did you feel about participating in religious activities?
28. Do you ever remember being ashamed of your parents (when they were poorly dressed, drunk, did not speak well, etc.)?
29. a. When you were punished by your parents, did they ever hurt you or leave marks?
    b. Were you physically abused? How did you feel about this? If you were physically abused, why did you think you were hurt? Was your mother or father drunk or high when they physically abused you?
30. Was there enough food when you were a child? Was there enough money for things needed?
31. Do you remember having fun as a child? Was there enough money for having fun? Did you at times feel "bought off"—in other words, given money when you really wanted to be hugged and praised?
32. Did your family move much from place to place? How did you feel? How did this affect your having friends?
33. Did your mother or father use drugs or alcohol? How did this affect how they related to you?
34. Were your parents divorced? If so, how old were you when that happened? Who did you then live with? At that age how did you explain to yourself what caused the divorce? Did you feel responsible? Did you side with one parent or the other and over the years who did you live with? Did you switch back and forth? When and why did this occur? Did you feel caught in the middle of their anger toward each other?
35. Were you ever in a foster family?
36. Did your mother or father act in ways that caused you to feel guilty or feel that you were not worthwhile? How do you think they did this?
37. Were there periods of your growing up when you felt close to your mother and father, and how did this change at different ages?
38. Did your family do things together or did everyone go their own way?
39. How much time did you spend with your family?
40. Did your family care about what you did or didn't do?
41. Write down any other memories of your family life, especially those times that were painful or sad. Now write down memories of any happy times.

My School Life

1. Write down what you remember about when you first went to school and how you felt (do you remember crying or being homesick and missing your mother)? Try to remember each grade in school and write down what you remember about each grade, what kind of grades you received, who was the teacher and how you felt about her or him, whether you did or didn't have friends in that class. Did you have any fights? Did you try and do well or did you not care?
2. What did you become frustrated with? What did you do that made you feel embarrassed or ashamed? What special interests did you have? Were they also the things that you did well?
3. Did you participate in physical education? Did you play any sports? How did you feel about these activities?
4. In each grade how did you behave (did you try to be funny, cause problems, work hard, or become the teacher's pet)? Did other students pick on you?
5. Did you ever repeat a grade or get "left back"? If you did, write why this took place and how you felt about it. Were you teased or did you get into fights over this? Did you ever skip a grade? If so, how did you feel about that? Were you ever in special education classes? Did you get individual help? How often (one hour a week, one hour a day)? For what class? Did you understand why you got this help and how did you feel about it? Were you teased?
6. Were you ever told or did you think that you had a learning disability? If so, what did that mean to you? How did you feel about it? How did your parents react to it? How did the teachers treat you about it?
7. Did you have difficulty concentrating? Were you considered hyperactive? How did teachers and others react to this? Were you ever put on medicine to help you concentrate? If so, how did you feel? Did the medicine help you to do better in school? Were you teased by the other children? Did you feel that you were stupid or something was wrong with your brain?
8. Were you considered a tough guy or girl in school?
9. Did you change from being shy to being considered tough and cool?
10. Were you ever suspended from school? Why?
11. If you dropped out of school, whose decision was this? Why did you drop out? Would you do it again?
12. Did you ever cheat in school? How often? Why did you cheat? How did it make you feel?
13. What things in school did you feel good about? Did you ever volunteer for extra activities? What were those?
14. How did you feel when report cards came out? Did you ever hide your card or try to change the grades because you were embarrassed by them? Did you feel that you were smart, stupid, had good ideas or dumb ideas? Did you have trouble solving problems?

15. Did you feel you could do better in school but just didn't know how or didn't want to because you were so frustrated or angry?
16. Were you ever sent to the principal or a counselor because of discipline problems? Describe what happened and how you felt.
17. What other activities, such as music lessons or dancing lessons, were you involved in during your school years? Did you feel successful at them? Were they fun or stressful?

My Worries, Anxieties, and Fears

1. As a child do you remember being afraid when you were alone? Did you miss your mother or worry that something had happened to her when you were away?
2. Were you afraid of the dark?
3. Were you afraid of bigger or tougher children and were you afraid to stand up for yourself and get into fights? Were you afraid not to fight because you would be considered a "wimp"?
4. Did things your parents told you make you afraid? Did they tell you that bad things would happen to you if you did not behave?
5. What things were you afraid to do? What did other children say about your fears? Could you tell someone, your mother, father, or a friend, that you were afraid of something?
6. Were you worried about how you looked? Did you worry about your face, body, or how you dressed? Did you think you looked ugly or strange or different? Write about these feelings. Were there any parts of you that you thought looked good and were proud of?
7. Were you afraid of your mother's reaction to anything you said or did? Are you still afraid?
8. Were you afraid of your father's reaction to anything you said or did? Are you still afraid?
9. What do you worry about now (money, success, how you look, what others think of you, that you will be teased over something you did, etc.)? Do you worry about making mistakes or being wrong about something?
10. Do you worry about getting hurt, that you will die, that something bad will happen to you, that you will have bad luck, that someone will hurt you?
11. Do you worry about winning or beating others at something? Why?
12. Do you worry that you will be successful, because then success will always be expected of you?
13. List all your present fears. What is your biggest fear at present?
14. Do you remember times when you had difficulty falling asleep because you were worried about something? What were you worried about at the time?

15. Were you afraid of roller coasters and going on fast rides?
16. Are you afraid of flying in airplanes?
17. Did you do the opposite and take risks to prove that you weren't afraid of doing things?

My Image—With Others and Myself

1. Did you have friends as a child? Did you have friends in the middle school years? Do you have friends now? What kind of friends? Have you changed friends or avoided close friends? Have you had special close friends? What kind of a friend are you to them?
2. Can other people depend on you? Do you come through for them? Has this changed over the years?
3. Do you change friends suddenly because you like someone better?
4. Do you gossip about others?
5. Have you betrayed a friend's secret by telling it to others?
6. Have you dropped any friends because you did not like how they looked or acted or because they were not cool enough?
7. Do you say things just to impress other people?
8. Has anybody ever said they felt used by you? Did you use them?
9. Do your friends think you are honest or dishonest? Why?
10. Why have you ended friendships? Do you ever end friendships quickly when you think they might not like you as much?
11. Are you cold and uncaring to friends?
12. Do you argue a lot with people?
13. Do you always consider yourself right and prefer to be only with friends who agree with you?
14. Do you have to prove to others how tough or cool you are?
15. Do you ever feel superior to others? Why (more brains, money, better neighborhood, the right skin color, hair color)? Are you covering up feelings of being inferior?
16. Do you think you are a big shot?
17. How do you compare yourself to others? Do you think you are more talented?
18. Are you jealous of others? Why?
19. Do you think you are inferior to others? Why?
20. Do you think others are smarter, have more money, look better, fit in better?
21. Are you always in competition with others?
22. Do you look at everything by comparing that you are one up or one down with others?
23. Do you make fun of others?
24. Do others make fun of you?

25. Are you a leader? Do you tell others what to do?
26. Do you decide what the plans are and who will be included?
27. Are you a follower? Do you do what others tell you to do?
28. Are you shy and anxious with other people? Have you always been like that?
29. How do you feel about others who may not have been as fortunate as you or don't have as much as you?
30. Are you tough on the outside but scared and feel like a wimp on the inside?
31. Do you consider yourself lucky or unlucky in life?
32. In what ways do you consider yourself lucky or unlucky in life?
33. When you get up in the morning and look in the mirror, how do you feel about what you see and who you are?
34. Do you try to con yourself that you feel differently about yourself than you really do? Describe how you fool yourself.
35. Do you complain to others and tell them how difficult life is for you?
36. Do you brag to others and tell them how great you are?
37. What are your good points?
38. What do you consider your weaknesses and bad points?
39. What has your mother thought of you as a child, a teenager, and after you began using drugs or alcohol?
40. Write about what your father has thought of you.
41. What do you feel good about that you have done or achieved (good grades, a good football game, good looking, etc.)?
42. Write about things that have made you feel embarrassed and ashamed.
43. Do you still have those feelings? Why?
44. Write about what kind of group of friends you have connected with. Does that group make you feel more secure or give you a particular image?

My Sexuality (No Names, Please!)

For Boys

1. As a young child what sort of things turned you on in a sexual way?
2. How old were you when you first masturbated? Were you ever caught and how did you feel about it? What were you told about masturbation by parents or friends? Did you ever masturbate in a group?
3. What other sexual things did you try out as a child?
4. Did you "play doctor" with girls or other boys?
5. Do you remember seeing your mother or father nude? How did you feel about that?
6. Did you ever see or hear when your parents were having sex? How did you feel?
7. Did you worry that you wouldn't become a real man or were too feminine?
8. Were you turned on when you looked at other boys? Did you do sexual things with other boys your own age? Were you ever sexually involved with older boys or adult men?
9. What did you think about or picture in your mind when you masturbated as a child and as a teenager?
10. In gym class or the restroom, how did you feel when you were around other boys who seemed more developed than you? Were you embarrassed by your body? Were you teased about your body?
11. Puberty begins when your penis and voice change and you develop hair in your genital area. Did you develop later than other boys? How did it make you feel?
12. Did you develop earlier than other boys and how did that make you feel?
13. Did you feel bad or guilty about your sexual feelings or body development? Were you ever sexually abused as a child or teenager? How did you feel? Did you tell anybody?
14. Did you have erections? Were you embarrassed or teased when they would occur in school or when out with friends?
15. How did you feel about your first sexual experience? Did you have sexual intercourse? How old were you and did you feel guilty, ashamed, proud, etc.? Were you pressured into doing it?
16. Write about your first girlfriend and later girlfriends. Did you fall head over heels in love or were you very cautious? Did you ever hurt your girlfriend emotionally or physically?
17. Did you use birth control when having sex? Did you use condoms or did you depend on the girl using something like pills? Did you just not worry that she might get pregnant?
18. Have you ever gotten a girl pregnant? What happened? Did she lose the baby, have an abortion, or have the baby? Tell how you felt about it.

19. Were you only concerned with how many girls you could have sex with and kept score? Did you brag to others to try and impress them?
20. Have you ever raped somebody or have you been raped?
21. Have you used sex to punish or reward someone?
22. Have you been afraid that girls would not be interested in you?
23. Do you have sexual feelings for other boys? How do you feel about this?
24. Do you have sexual feelings for children? Have you ever acted on these feelings?
25. Write about what your sex life is today and how you feel about it. Do you think it is "normal"? What about it do you consider not normal?
26. Write about love. Was love part of your having sex?
27. Write about romantic and sexual relationships that made you unhappy, angry, anxious, frustrated or feel used. What do you relate these feelings to?
28. Describe any sexual activity that you have done that you consider perverted or abnormal.
29. Write about sexual and romantic relationships that made you feel happy, cared about, and valued.

Continue now with the section titled My Actions on page 49.

My Sexuality (No Names, Please!)

For Girls

1. What do you remember as a young child about having sexual feelings? What things made you feel sexy?
2. Write about when you first masturbated, how you felt and what you thought about.
3. What sexual things did you do as a child? Did you "play doctor"?
4. Did you do sexual things with other girls your own age? Were you ever sexually involved with older girls or adult women?
5. Did you have sexual contact with your father, a brother, or another relative?
6. Write about when you saw your parents nude and how you felt.
7. Write about when you saw or heard your parents having sex and how it made you feel.
8. Write about how you felt about your body? Did you feel you were attractive, sexy, ugly, or embarrassed?
9. Were you ever sexually abused as a child or teenager? How did you feel? Did you get help or tell anybody?
10. How did you feel when you first began to menstruate? How did your mother or father react to this? Did you feel embarrassed, proud, ashamed? Where were you when it first happened?
11. Puberty begins when your breasts begin to develop and you develop hair in your genital area. Did you develop early? Tell about how you felt about that.
12. Did you develop sexually late? How did that affect how you felt about yourself? Were you teased?
13. Did your family talk about sex? In what way?
14. What did you think about the sexual relationship between your mother and father?
15. Tell about the first time you had sexual intercourse and how you felt. Did you feel pressured into it?
16. Write about whether you used birth control. Did you worry about becoming pregnant?
17. Have you ever been pregnant? If you were, did you lose the baby, have an abortion, or have the baby? How do you feel about this?
18. If you have ever had an abortion, write about how you felt. How did you feel about yourself? How did you feel toward the baby's father? Did he support you through this or just leave you?
19. Have you ever used sex to attract boys? Have you ever used sex to hurt boys?
20. What was your reputation in school?
21. Have you ever been raped? Write about what happened. How did you feel, how has it affected you, and how have you tried to cope with this?
22. Have you ever used sex to punish or reward someone?

23. Have you used sex to avoid loneliness?
24. Have you been afraid that you are not attractive sexually?
25. What do you think about how you make love now? Do you think it is "normal"?
26. Do you have sexual feelings for other girls? How do you feel about this?
27. What things have you done that you felt were sexually abnormal?
28. Write about what you think love is.
29. Have you been in love with a person who is uncaring and cold? Why did you stay with him?
30. Have you ever been physically abused in any of your romantic relationships? How did you feel about this?
31. Have you ever felt used or abused?
32. Have you stayed in relationships because you did not want to hurt the boy's feelings or because of your insecurity?
33. Write about any sexual and romantic relationships that made you feel unhappy, anxious, frustrated, or embarrassed.
34. Write about any sexual and romantic relationships that made you feel happy, cared about, and valued.

Continue now with the next section, titled My Actions.

My Actions

1. Did you lie as a child? Why? Did it help you get out of trouble? Were you caught? Did people believe you? Did you continue lying? Were you punished? How?
2. Describe the first time you stole anything. What did you steal as a child? What did you steal as a teenager?
3. Were you given an allowance? How did you behave about money? Did you save your money or did you spend it as soon as you received it? Did you spend it on yourself or on others?
4. Did you ever buy alcohol or drugs with money that was supposed to be used for something else (clothes, books, or school supplies)?
5. Did you destroy your own things or other people's property?
6. Were you a bully or a tough guy? Did you get into fights? Did you start them? Did you take up for yourself? Were you encouraged to do this by your mother or father?
7. Did you have tantrums and angry outbursts? Do you still have them?
8. Did you break rules and laws? How did you feel about it?
9. Write about the illegal things you have done. Have you ever used a fake ID? Have you ever tried to cash checks that weren't yours? Did you steal money from others or use credit cards of your parents or other people?
10. How do you feel about driving? Do you show off when driving? Do you drive drunk? Does a car show how brave and tough you are?
11. List any medical illnesses that you have had. Did you use them to avoid doing things you were supposed to do? Did you get attention when you were sick?
12. Did you pretend to be sick at times when you weren't? Why?

My Jobs

1. What chores did you have at home? Did you do them or avoid them?
2. Did you ever have a part-time or full-time job?
3. Describe the jobs you have had. Describe whether you liked or disliked these jobs.
4. What did your boss think of you?
5. Were you ever fired from a job? If so, describe when and why.
6. Did you work for extra spending money or did you work to help support yourself or your family?

My Summary

1. List what you are *still* angry about.
2. List what you are *still* sad about.
3. List what you are *still* guilty about.
4. What have been your *best* experiences in life?
5. What have been your *worst* experiences in life?
6. Write down the secrets about yourself that you've thought you would never tell.
7. Can you begin to believe that you can be a worthwhile person?

Step 5

Admitted to God, to ourselves, and to another human being the exact nature of our wrongs.

Step 5 involves sharing your Fourth Step with another person. In Step 4 you wrote down all the terrible and hurtful things that were done to you in your life and that you did to others. You identified all the feelings of hate, guilt, sadness, and fear. Now you need to tell them to someone you can trust.

The person with whom you do your Fifth Step must be a very special person. A recovering person who is or may become your sponsor or a special staff member is usually best. Write down the first name of the person you would like to do your Fifth Step with: ______________________.

Check whether this person meets the following conditions:

1. Can you trust him or her with *all* of your secrets? _____ Yes _____ No.
2. Won't be hurt or angry by what you say? _____ Yes _____ No.
3. Is a recovering member of AA or NA who understands the importance of this step and has done it himself or herself? _____ Yes _____ No.
4. You won't meet this person in your everyday home, work, or school environment? _____ Yes _____ No.

You need all Yes answers to go ahead. Step 5 will require at least two hours and often up to five or six hours. Once you have completed the Fourth Step, you need to do the Fifth Step as soon as possible. Push yourself to do it before leaving the hospital or residential program. Now schedule the date __________, and the time __________.

Let someone else hear your story and forgive you.

Then you can forgive yourself *and go on to a new way of life.*

Continuing Recovery

Congratulations! You've completed the first Five Steps of AA/NA and are in recovery. By now you should like yourself better, be more honest, and care about yourself and others. Now the goal is to continue your recovery after this intensive hospital or residential part of your program.

Remember—you're better but *not* cured. Chemical dependency (addiction) is a life-long disorder, and you must keep working your program to keep off alcohol or drugs. The addict part of you continues to be present and must be kept in check by the healthy part of you which works your program. The first Five Steps must continue to be reworked. You must recognize *every day* that you are an addict and cannot use any alcohol or drugs (the First Step). You must still complete Steps 6 through 12, which involve changing your behavior, making amends, continuing your personal inventory, and enhancing your spirituality. Your aftercare program and sponsor will help you to continue your life-long recovery.

The following points are essential for your continued recovery. Check off this list frequently to make sure you are working your program.

1. Be thankful—for having a real life, for people who care about you, for being in treatment.
2. Work your Steps—work the First Step every day, rework Steps 2 through 5 as soon as possible, then begin on Steps 6 through 12.
3. Attend an AA/NA meeting every day.
4. Call your contacts and sponsor frequently.
5. Have meditative time with your Higher Power.
6. Continue your psychiatric care—see your therapist, take medications that have been medically prescribed.
7. Avoid contact with old friends who are still drinking or using drugs. Make new friends with people who are working good AA/NA programs.
8. No matter what—*Don't use any alcohol or drugs.*

Take Care!

Thoughts on Steps 6-12

Thoughts on Steps 6-12

Thoughts on Steps 6-12

Thoughts on Steps 6-12

Thoughts on Steps 6-12

Thoughts on Steps 6-12

Thoughts on Steps 6-12

Thoughts on Steps 6-12

1-882103-00-9